Cauldron Conversions

Cup	Oz	Tbsp	Tsp	ML
1	8	16	48	237
3/4	6	12	36	177
2/3	5	11	32	158
1/2	4	8	24	118
1/3	3	5	16	79
1/4	2	4	12	59
1/8	1	2	6	30
1/16	1/2	1	3	15
1/48	1/6	1/3	1	5

2 Cups = 1 Pint   4 Cups = 1 Quart

4 Quarts = 1 Gallon

May your cauldron
always be full

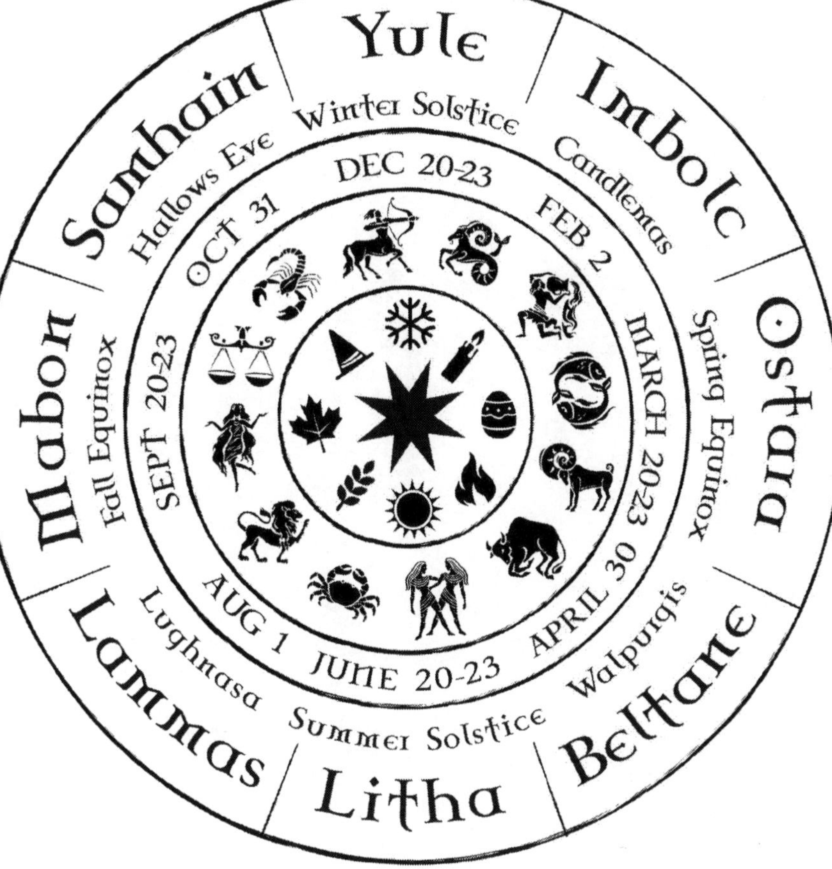

The Wheel of the Year is an ancient calendar based on the transition of the sun through the four seasons:

Spring Summer

Autumn Winter

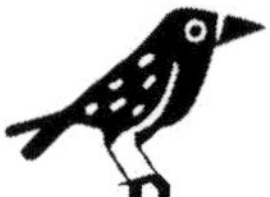

Recipe For:

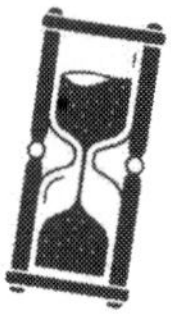

Prep Time: ____________ Temperature: ________

Cook Time: ____________ Serves: ____________

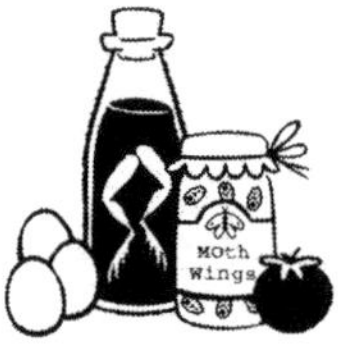

Ingredients

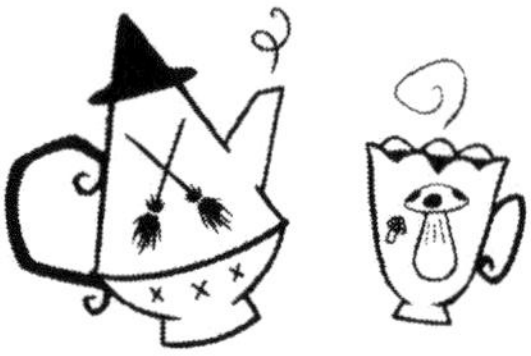

Directions

Notes

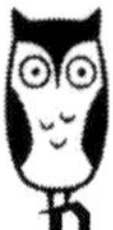

Recipe For:

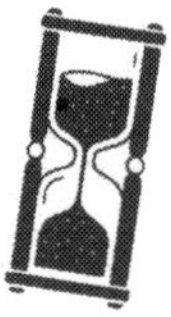

Prep Time: ____________ Temperature: ______

Cook Time: ____________ Serves: ____________

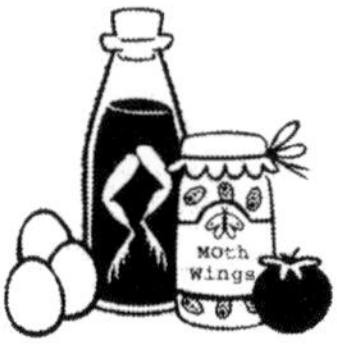

Ingredients

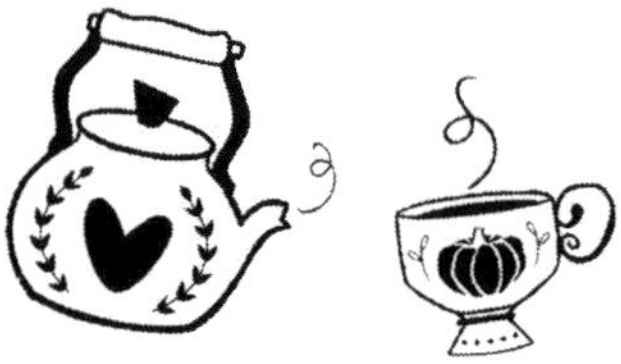

Directions

Notes

Recipe For:

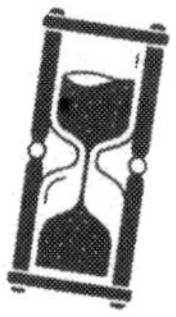

Prep Time: ____________ Temperature: ________

Cook Time: ____________ Serves: ____________

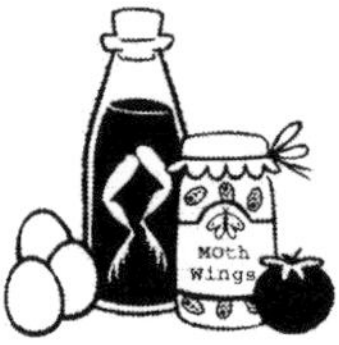

Ingredients

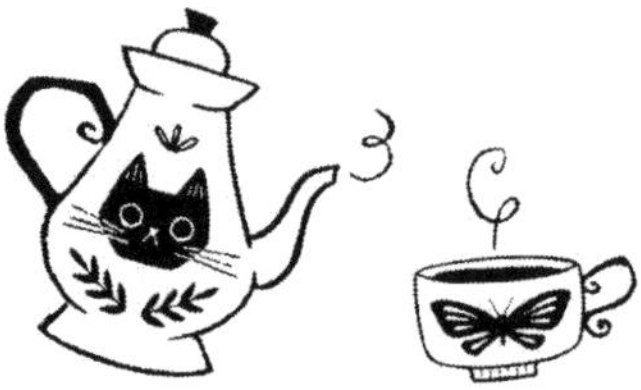

Directions

Notes

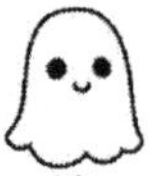

Recipe For:

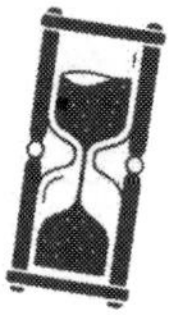

Prep Time: ________ Temperature: ________

Cook Time: ________ Serves: ________

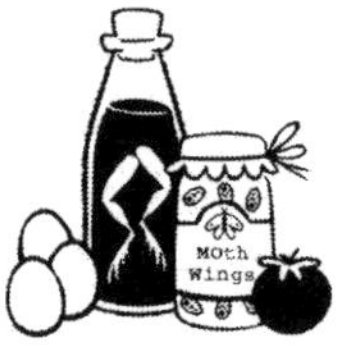

Ingredients

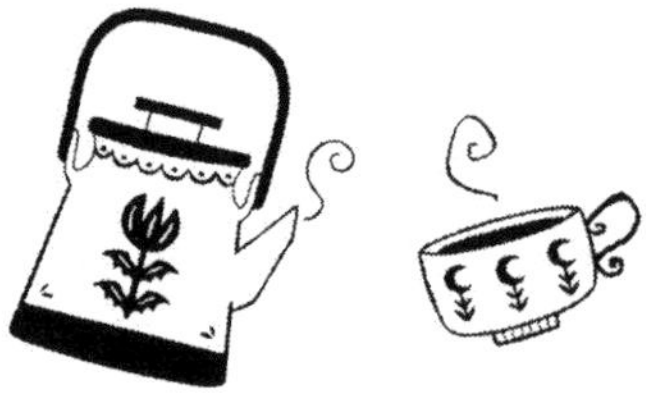

Directions

Notes

Recipe For:

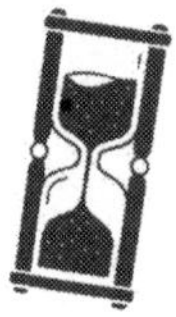

Prep Time: ____________ Temperature: ____________

Cook Time: ____________ Serves: ____________

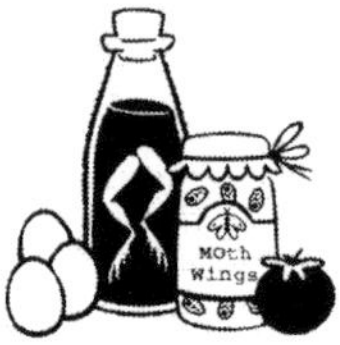

Ingredients

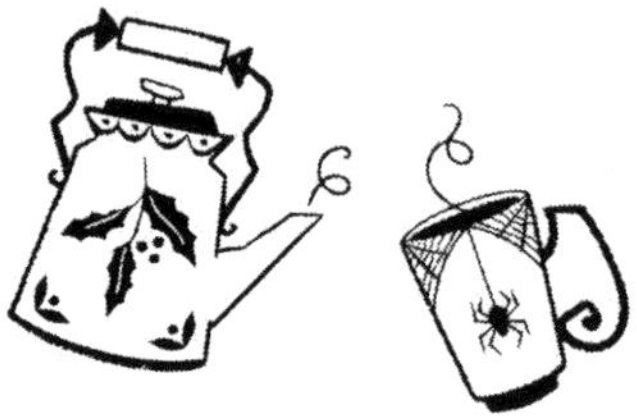

Directions

Notes

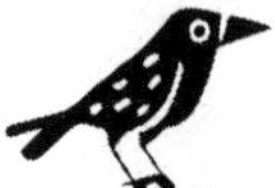

Recipe For:

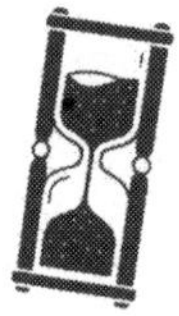

Prep Time: ____________ Temperature: ______

Cook Time: ____________ Serves: ____________

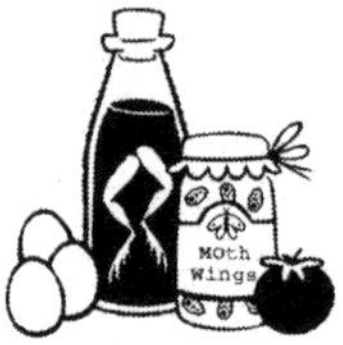

Ingredients

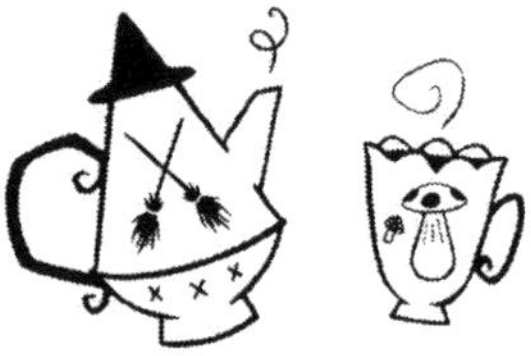

Directions

Notes

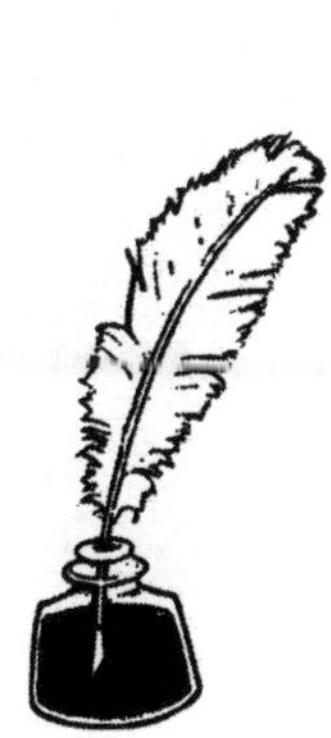

Recipe For:

Prep Time: ______ Temperature: ______

Cook Time: ______ Serves: ______

Ingredients

Directions

Notes

Recipe For:

Prep Time: ____________ Temperature: ________

Cook Time: ____________ Serves: ____________

Ingredients

Directions

Notes

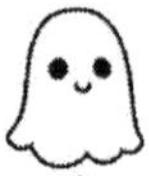

Recipe For:

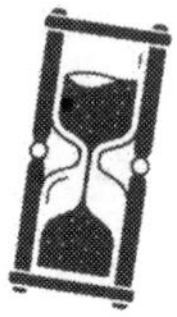

Prep Time: ________ Temperature: ________

Cook Time: ________ Serves: ________

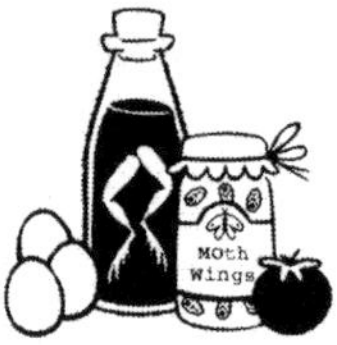

Ingredients

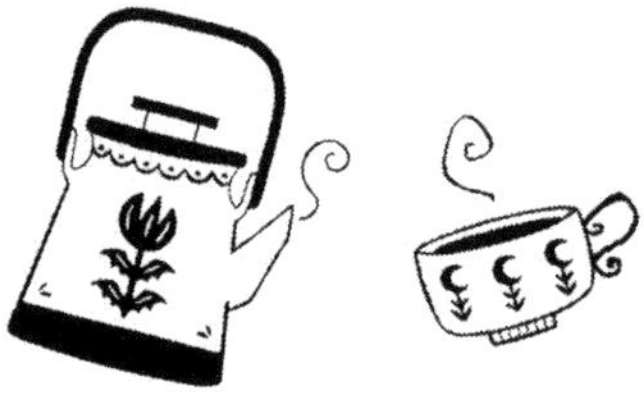

Directions

Notes

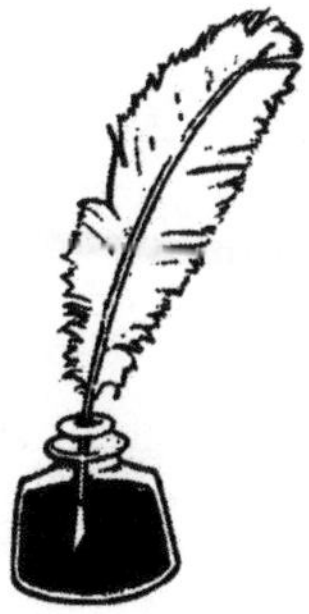

Recipe For:

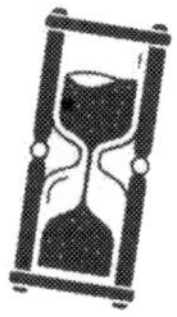

Prep Time: ____________ Temperature: ____________

Cook Time: ____________ Serves: ____________

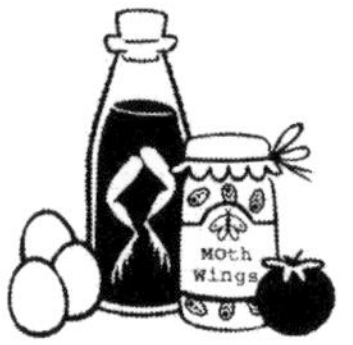

Ingredients

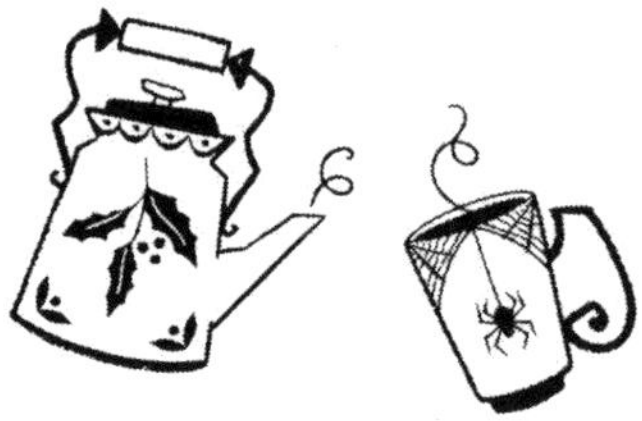

Directions

Notes

Recipe For:

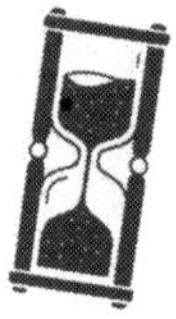

Prep Time: ______ Temperature: ______

Cook Time: ______ Serves: ______

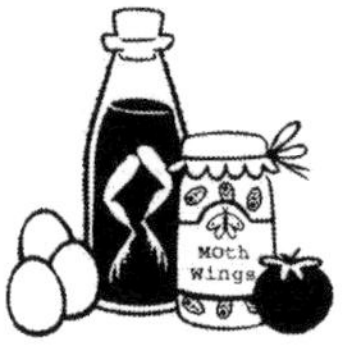

Ingredients

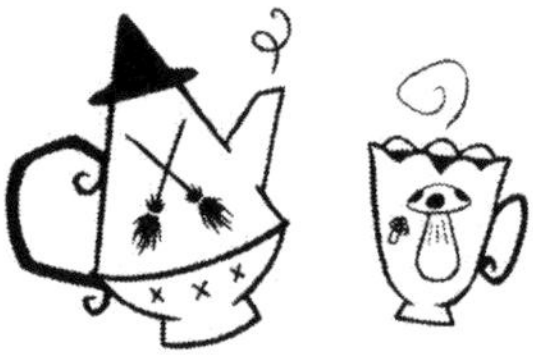

Directions

Notes

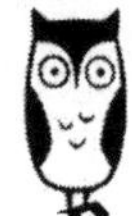

Recipe For:

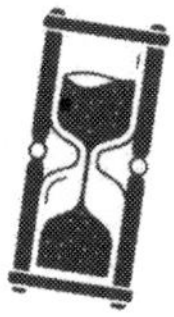

Prep Time: ________ Temperature: ________

Cook Time: ________ Serves: ________

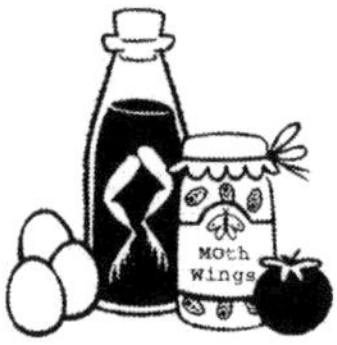

Ingredients

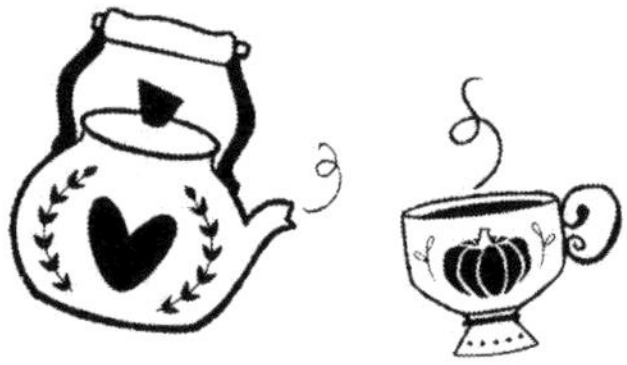

Directions

Notes

Recipe For:

Prep Time: ____________ Temperature: ____________

Cook Time: ____________ Serves: ____________

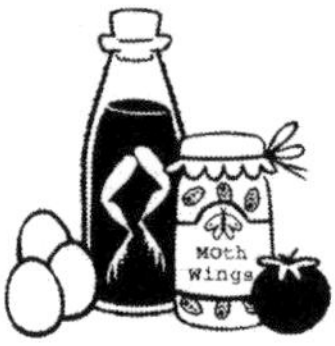

Ingredients

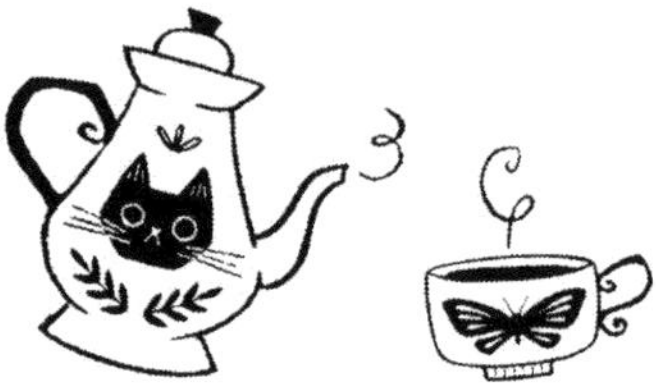

Directions

Notes

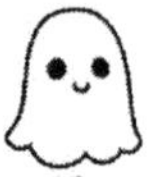

Recipe For:

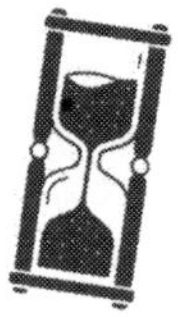

Prep Time: ________ Temperature: ________

Cook Time: ________ Serves: ________

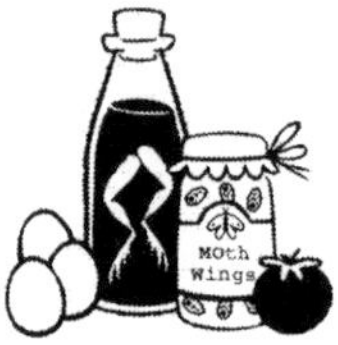

Ingredients

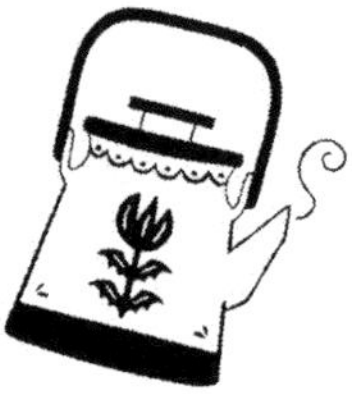

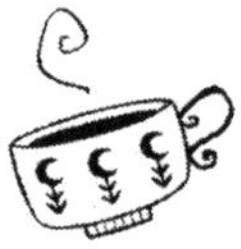

Directions

Notes

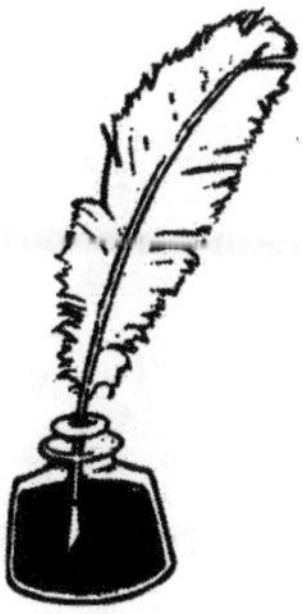

Recipe For:

Prep Time: ________ Temperature: ________

Cook Time: ________ Serves: ________

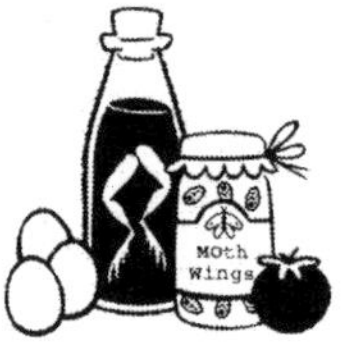

Ingredients

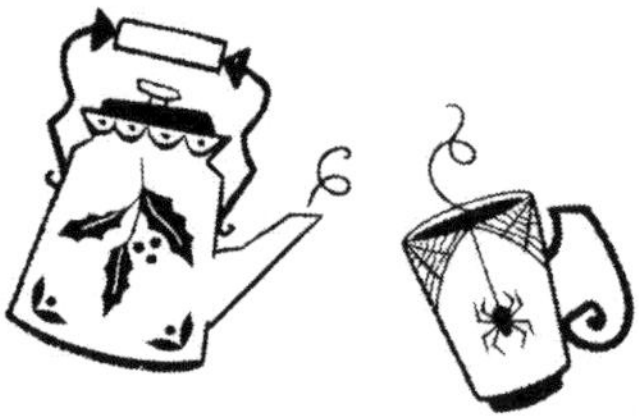

Directions

Notes

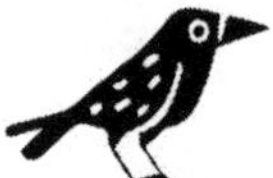

Recipe For:

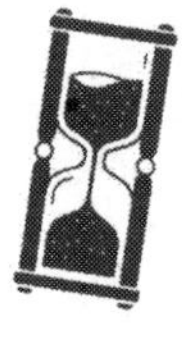

Prep Time: ______ Temperature: ______

Cook Time: ______ Serves: ______

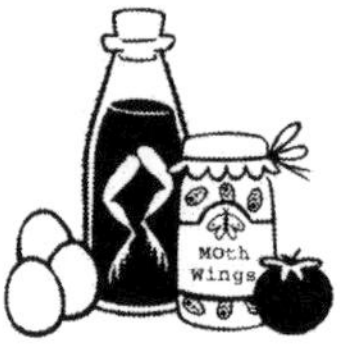

Ingredients

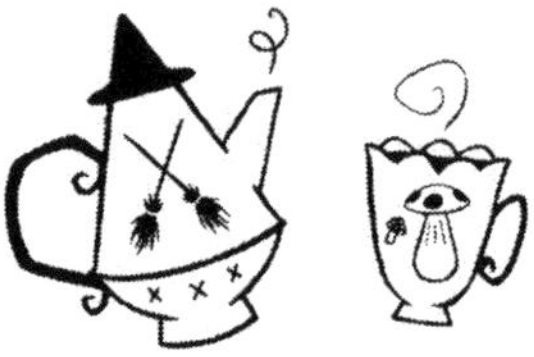

Directions

Notes

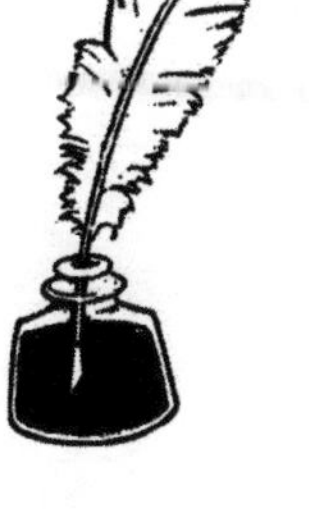

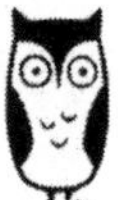

Recipe For:

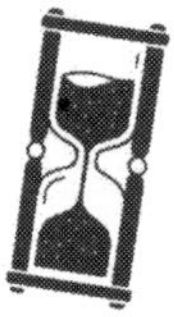

Prep Time: ________ Temperature: ________

Cook Time: ________ Serves: ________

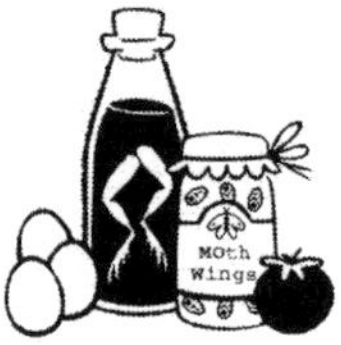

Ingredients

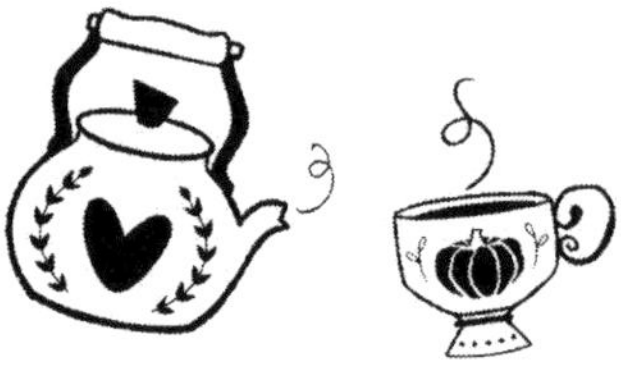

Directions

Notes

Recipe For:

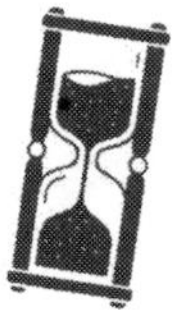

Prep Time: ____________ Temperature: ______

Cook Time: ____________ Serves: ____________

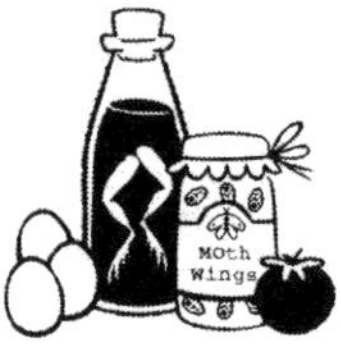

Ingredients

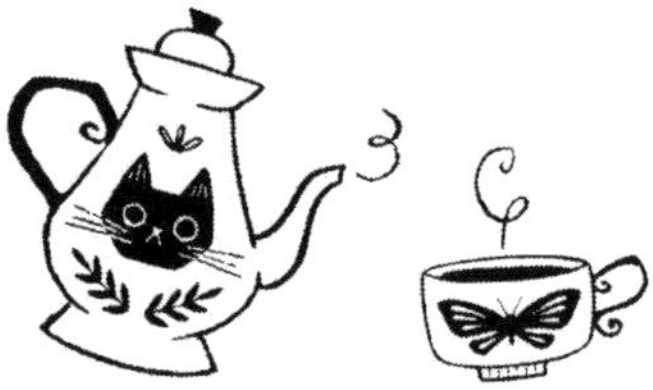

Directions

Notes

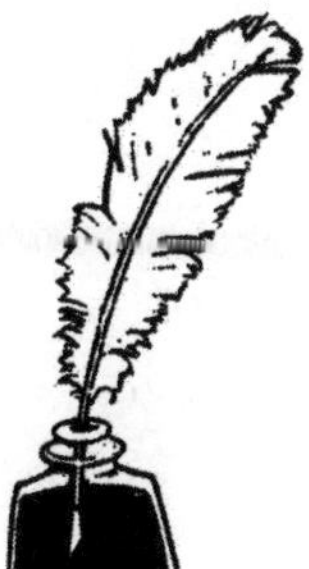

Published by Sketchy Pumpkin Books

The Sketchy Pumpkin LLC

2022 Chicago, IL USA

ISBN: 978-1-7350560-1-2

Made in the USA
Monee, IL
12 November 2026

7600adbe-1b87-44df-943a-716f010f59d0R01